SANITY IN VANITY

JOMYIR JINI

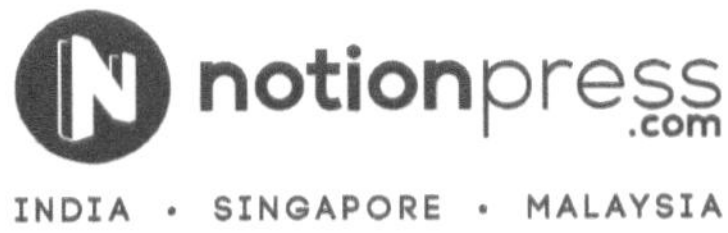

notionpress.com

INDIA • SINGAPORE • MALAYSIA

Notion Press

No.8, 3rd Cross Street
CIT Colony, Mylapore
Chennai, Tamil Nadu – 600004

First Published by Notion Press 2021
Copyright © Jomyir Jini 2021
All Rights Reserved.

ISBN 978-1-63873-503-8

Preface

The world is a shitty place to be alive today.

Was the world a better place when humans had to walk for days in search of food and fodder or was it a better place when pizza was not available at doorstep yet?

We will never know.

For the comparison to be logically correct, we need someone who've lived through all of this (now would be a good time for the Vampires to come out of their hiding).

Where am I going with all this? Is that no matter how shitty the situation is, it's your situation.

Own your shit!

Acknowledgement

Thank you,
My brain cells that have been bearing the brunt of thousands of electrical impulses running in several directions, all at once.
Thank you,
My heart muscles for pumping everyday for the last 25 years, sometimes void, but still pumping.
Thank you.

Smoking kills and so does overthinking.

Take this opportunity to thank yourself for battling yet another day!

love

is

but

not

just

kisses

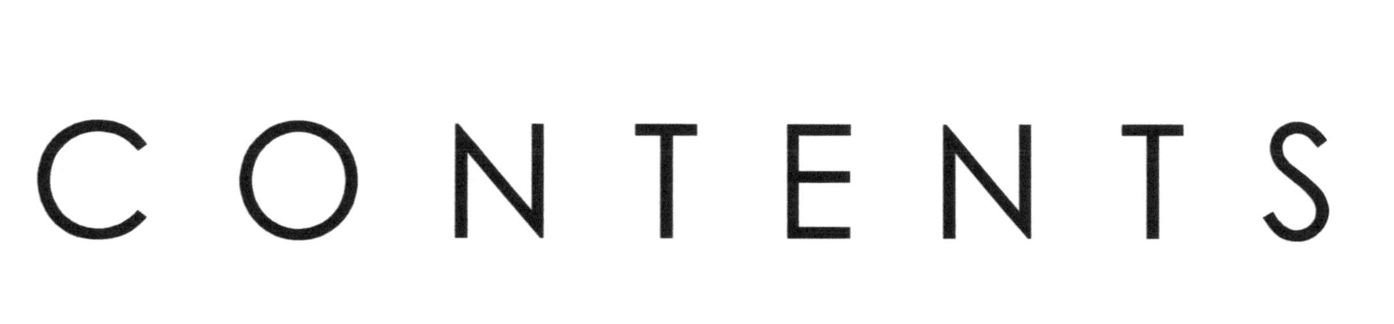

CONTENTS

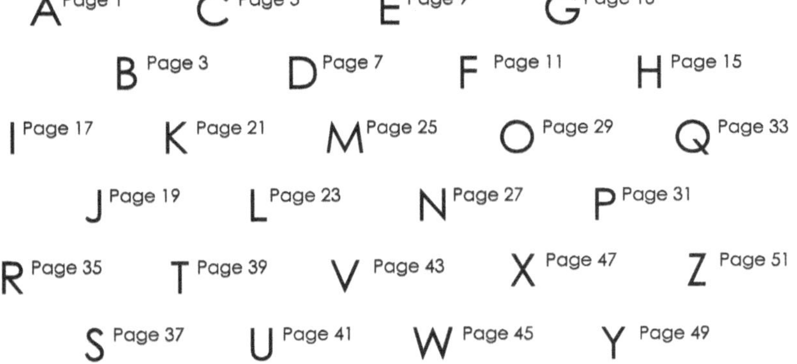

shadows on the walls

towards me it crawls

i tell it to you

shadows on the walls

towards me it crawls

inching closer day by day

shadows on the walls

towards me it crawls

it settled on me today

shadows on the walls

towards me it crawls

i screamed a mumbled-shush

shadows on the walls

towards me it crawls

wide awake i couldn't feel my legs

shadows on the walls

towards me it crawls

i fought and fought in vain

shadows on the walls

towards me it crawls

i let it, let it drain
shadows on the walls
towards me it crawls
and made friendship with
shadows on the walls
towards me it crawls
now i laugh at the disabled shadows
crawling on my walls
who cannot run
who cannot dance
shadows on the walls
i let it, let it crawl
for that is all it can do
shadows on the walls
it crawls

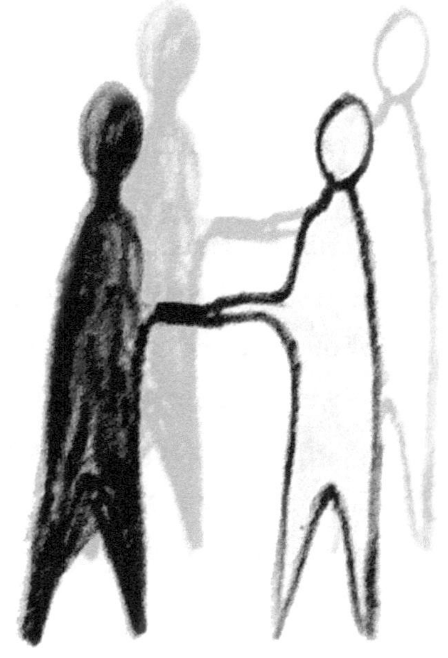

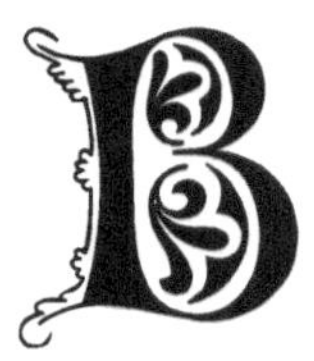

sometimes
more often than a normal
sometimes
a terrifi ed me
calms myself down

      it is an important art
      to stay alive

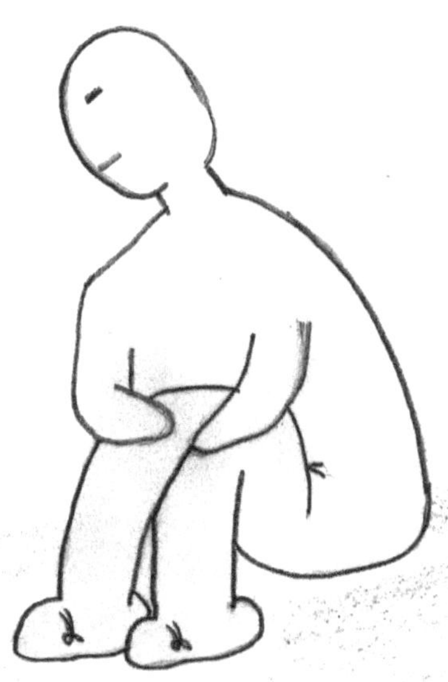

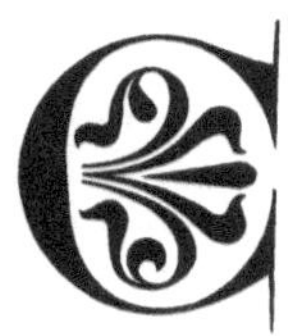

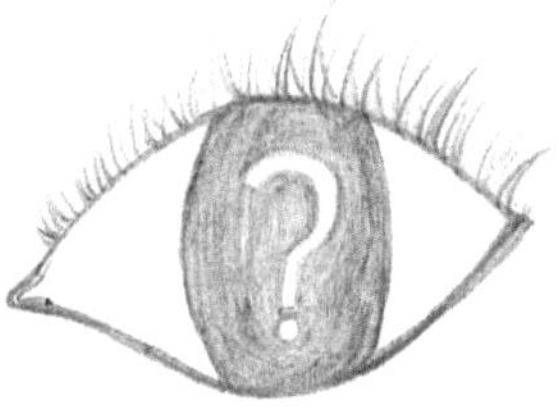

beauty

lies in the eyes of the beholder you say
isn't it time to question it's way?
why should your perception make me sway?

beauty

lies in the eyes of the beholder you say
may be, all that it really is
is all just a lie

beauty

lies in the eyes of the beholder
please don't say
i am beautiful
beautiful in ways
your eyes don't see
i am beautiful in many ways

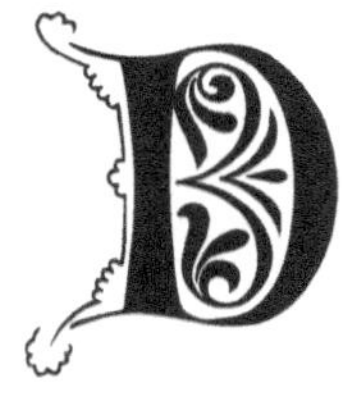

i waited upon the stars
as if it'll heal my scars
i waited upon the moon
hoping you'd return soon

i waited
i waited

i wish i had known
i am the sun on my own

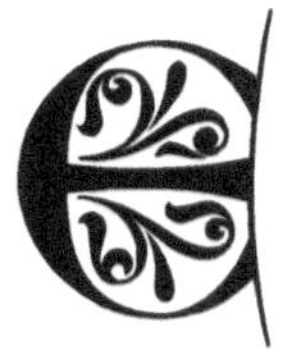

when you feel a lonely tinker
pointer, middle and ring fi nger
take them to your wrist
can you feel the resist?

      that is you

      beating for you

      fi rst for you

just for you

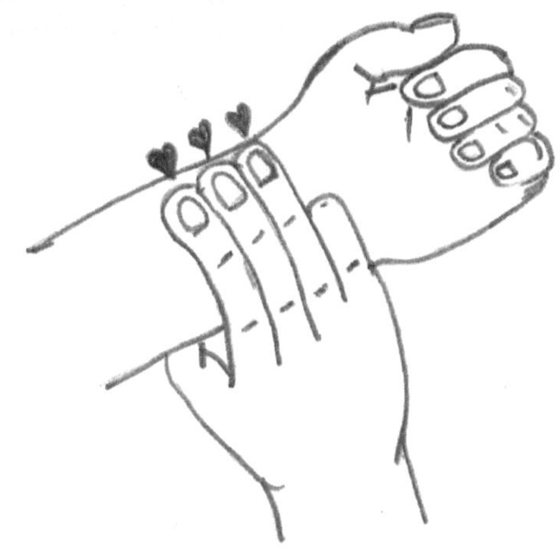

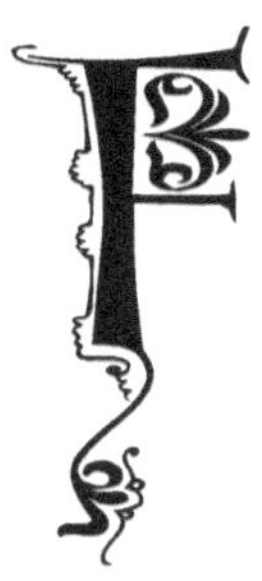

some days a struggle
to launch-pad
some days a struggle
to leave the bed
some days a victory
to ace the race
some days a victory
to face your face

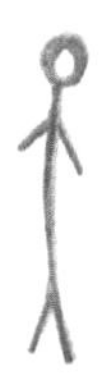

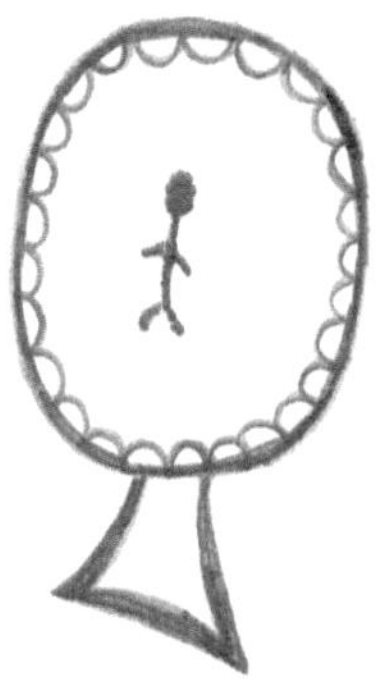

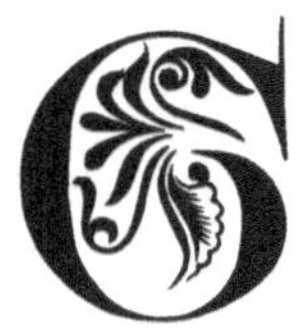

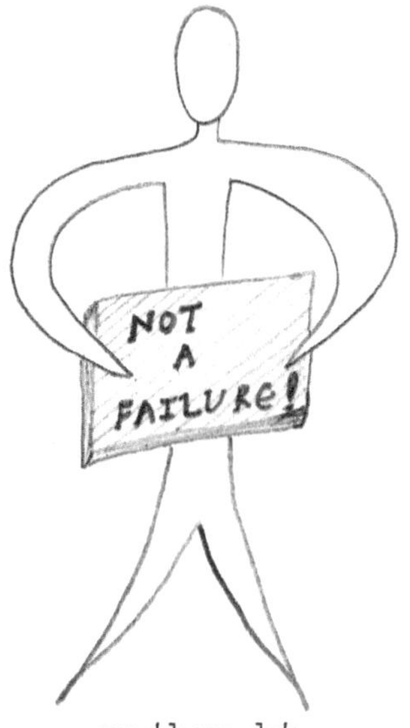

you thought
you could do it
you couldn't though
the task is
a failure
you are not
a failure
it's okay
you're okay

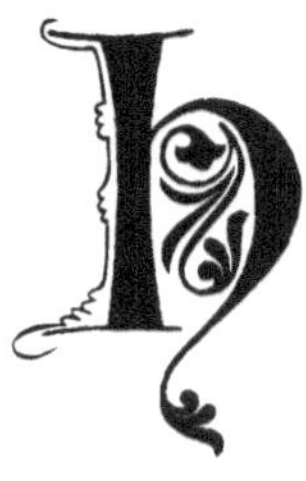

my mom knows
a different me
my dad knows
a different me
each sibling
yet other versions
you know
a different me
i know
a different me
and i've come to
embrace
all of me

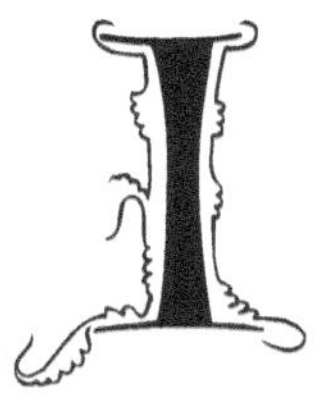

i've felt
mountains high
i've felt
oceans deep
in the dreams
that i dream
in the dreams
that i scream
lullabies that i sing
when it doesn't
stop to ring

eerieness blankets over
there is nothing to cover
in my dreams that i scream
have you had such a dream?

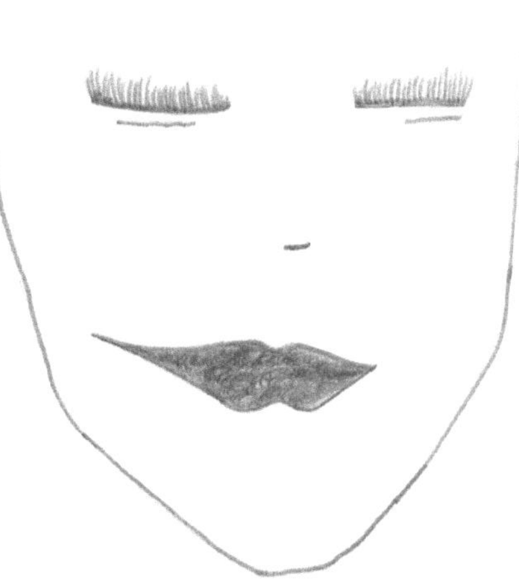

even then
in the midst
i wouldn't choose
those cut-wrists

oozing blood
tells a lie
world is a wreck
eye-for-an-eye

i've felt
mountains high
i've felt
oceans deep
in the dreams
that i dream
in my dreams
i still scream

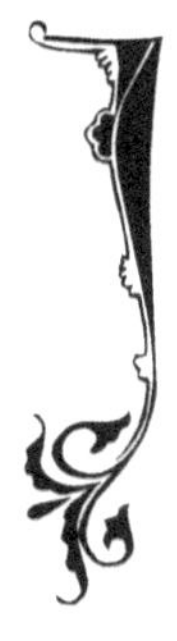

hello there!
fellow dear!
walking this trodden path
we meet at last
each hoping
to have outdone
each hoping
to far away, run
trapped
in this life's maze
at my own choices, amazed
i am treading down this path
don't know how long it will last

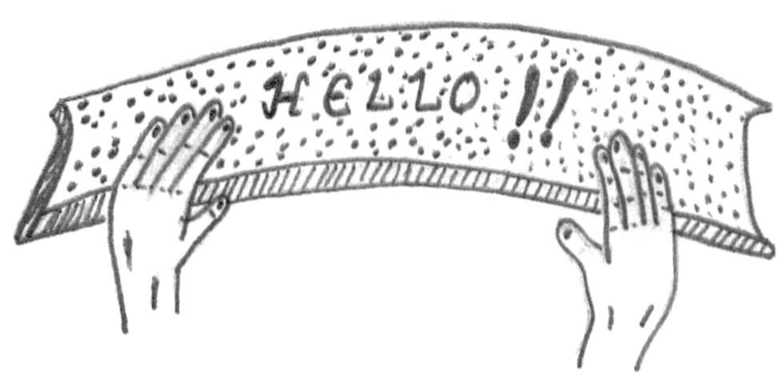

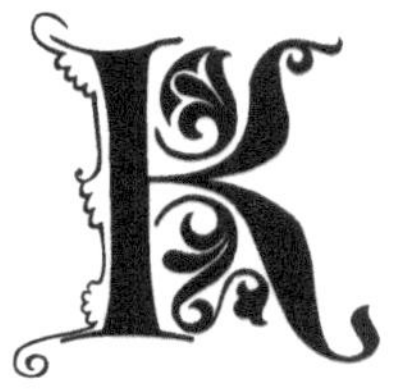

have you been there?

where words can't be heard
where colours can't be seen
where you bleed from within
your tears run dry
you try and try

try
i beg
please try

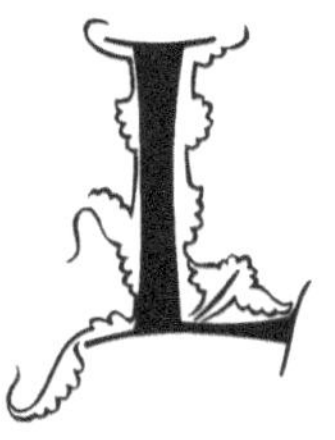

stumble
fumble
slip
trip
roll
fall
crawl
howl

soon
you'll reach
your stop

until then
you don't stop

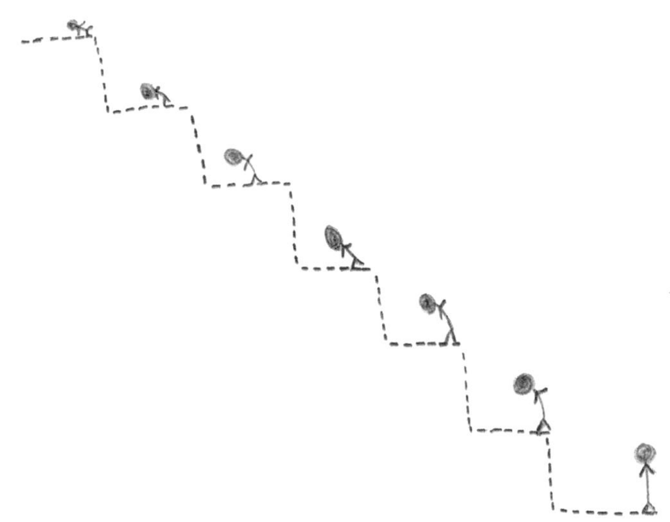

no less
not a mess
untamed
unashamed

at my pace
in my space
growing
slowly

slowly
growing

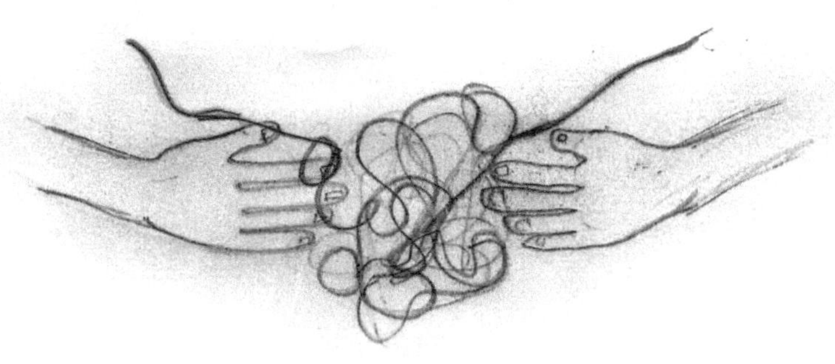

belong to a corner
this lame loner

pushed and pulled
ridiculed

hopping from hole to hole
hoping for role

you are your own hero
it all begins from zero

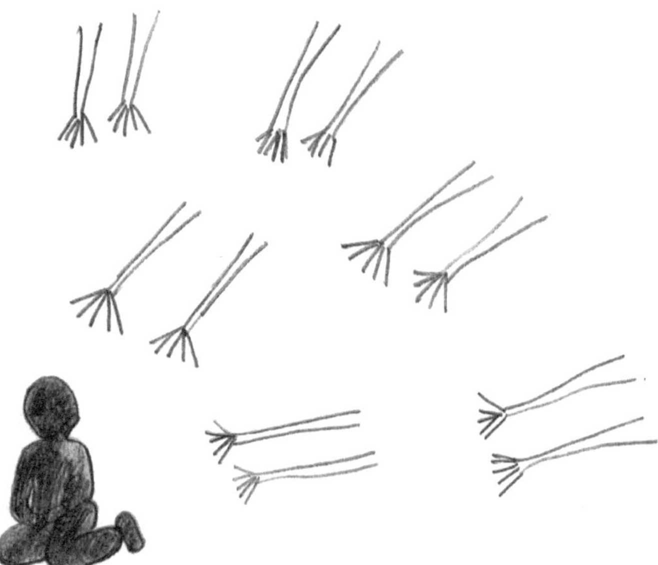

either too much
or too less
big booty
or small breasts
running away
or being chased
oh! this world
is surely
two-faced

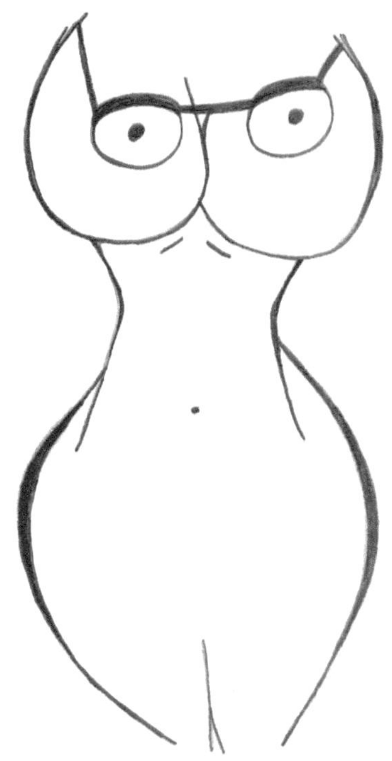

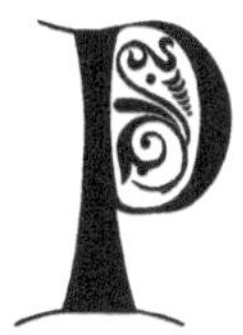

in life
there are many
firsts
in life
there are many
lasts

    there are first firsts
    and last firsts
    there are first lasts
    and last lasts
    and we'll
    never know
    when what

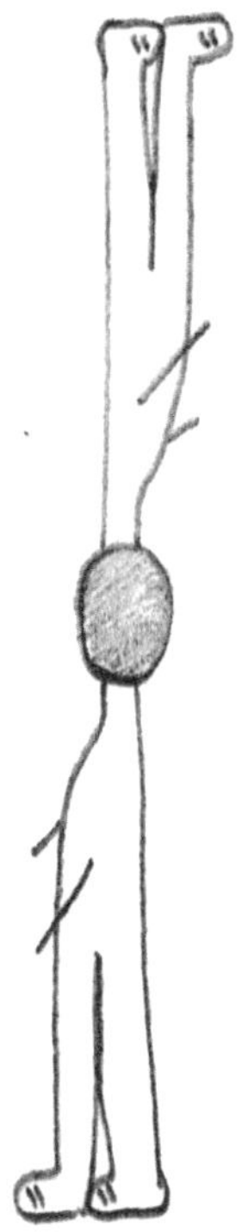

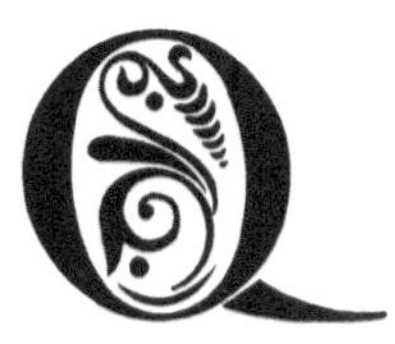

busy streets
half-hearted greets
everyone running
for end meets

we miss out

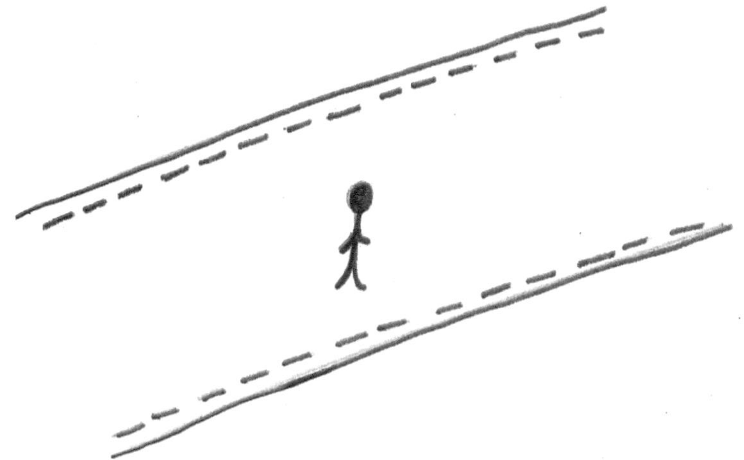

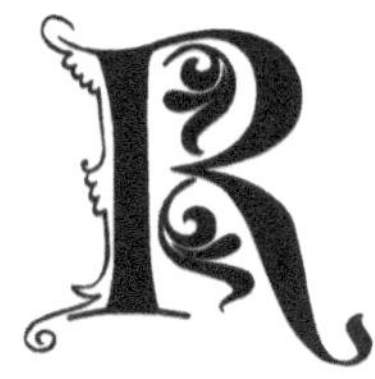

time and tide
wait for none

time
i have lost track of
a long time ago
tide
will eventually fall down
so
i
can
still
have a go

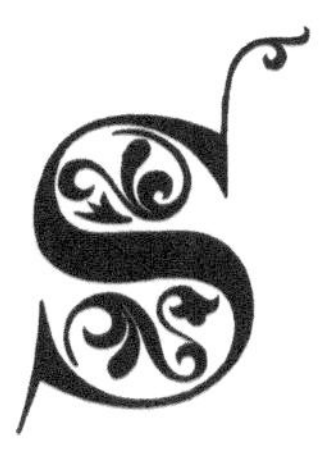

do you ever grow out of your insecurities
or is it made out of e l a s t i c s ?

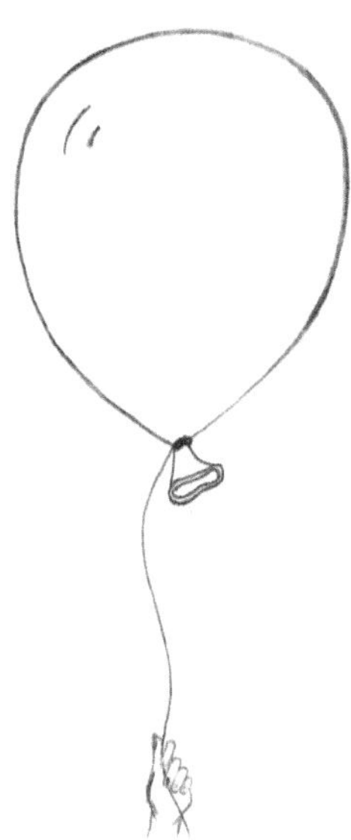

37

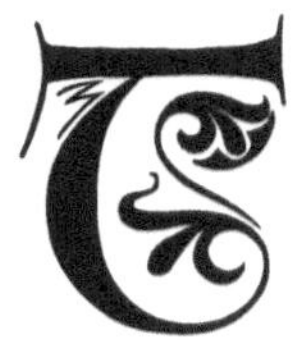

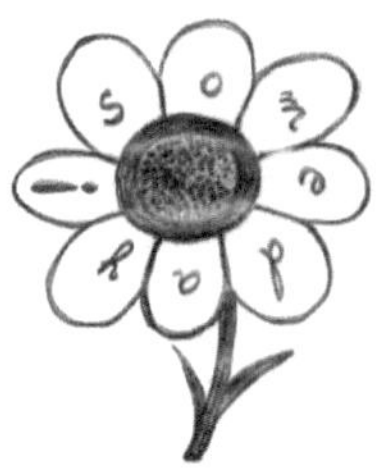

not ready yet to start
not ready yet to depart
not ready yet to talk
not ready yet to walk
not ready yet
someday

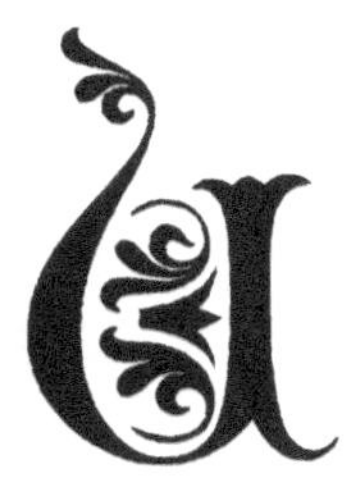

a stench in the air
refusing to clear
a lump in my throat
and a drowning boat
Oh! how to breathe
when buried deep

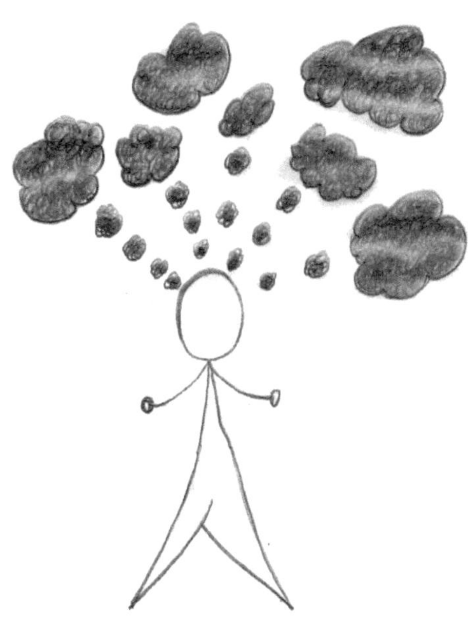

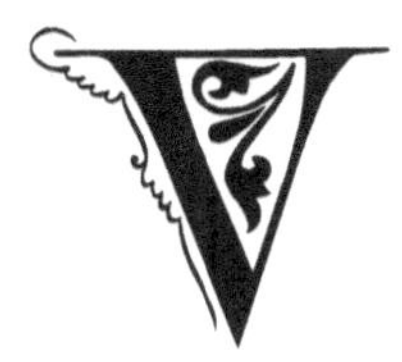

reach out, to see behind the curled lips
reach out, to listen to the unsaid
reach out, to help untangle
we're all a mess
some, messier
reach out

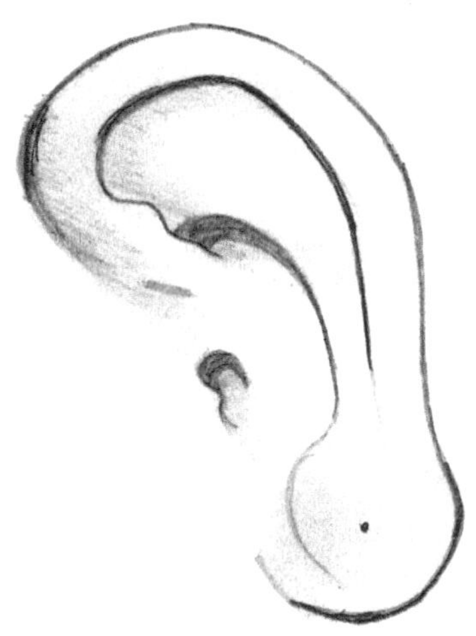

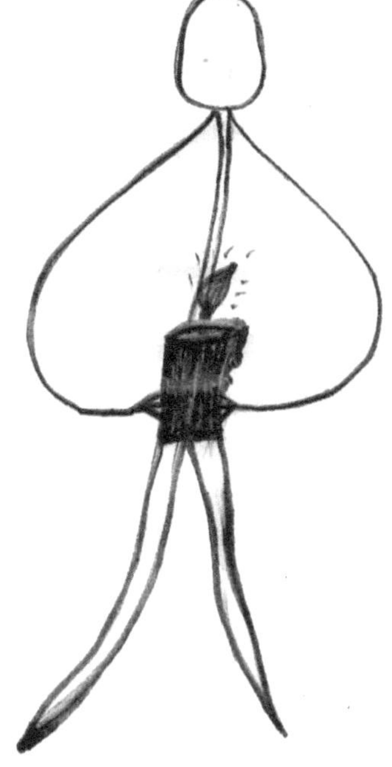

no
i don't understand

i don't understand
why i need a man

why you need a woman

     i hope
     you too
     you won't understand

     i hope you light your spark first
     kill your hunger; fill your thirst first
     though this world makes you sore
     i hope you stay strong, at your core

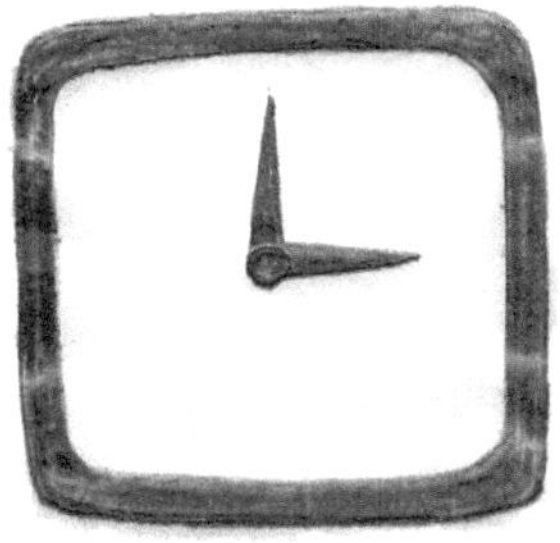

several set of eyes wide awake
several fears you cannot shake

we all have our 3 am moments

wrapped in this loneliness
you aren't a lone mess

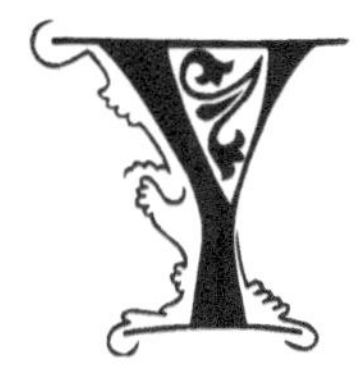

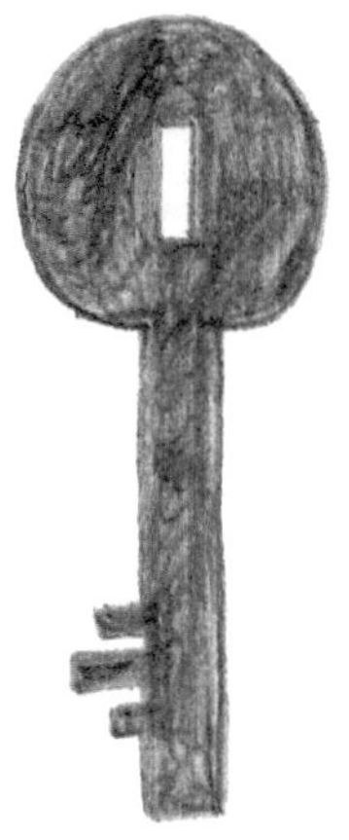

who has the key
to open you and see?
who has the key
to say, you're not free!
i hope you engage
in your little spree
who has the key
i hope your answer is

'i'

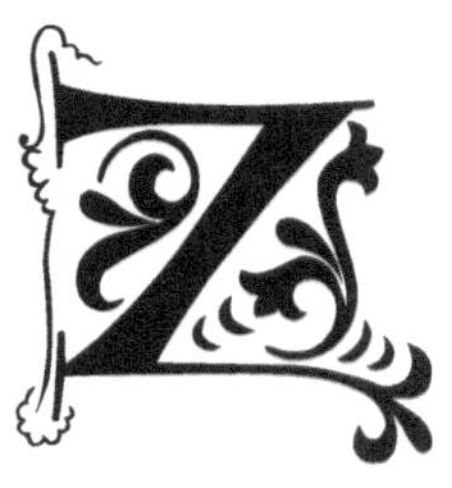

i've found my sanity
in my vanity
don't know what lies ahead
in my destiny
but in this moment
i choose to be mine
slippery like a slime
still, i choose to be mine

there's a fi re burning
insides of my stomach
churning
standing at this cross-road
with these life's load
bending by the burdens
bending at the weight
bending
not breaking

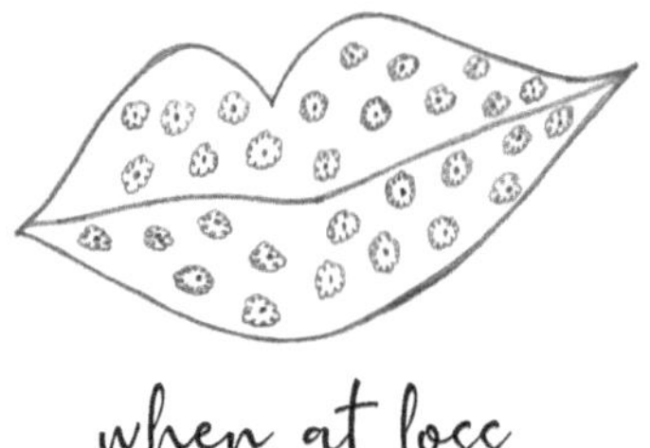

when at loss
take a pause

www.ingramcontent.com/pod-product-compliance
Lightning Source LLC
Chambersburg PA
CBHW031427250726
48656CB00002B/859